THE PREGNAN ___IDE
FOR FIRST-TIME DADS

*The Ultimate Handbook
with Everything You Need to Know
to Become the Best New Father*

Samuel Collins

0

Table of Contents

4

Introduction

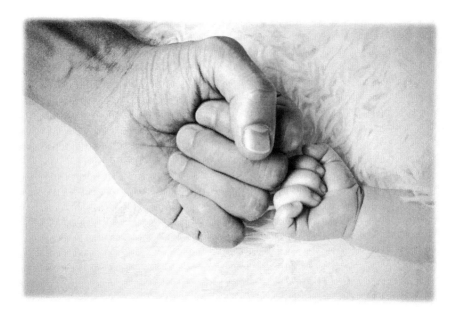

The nine-month journey that awaits from the time your partner falls pregnant is in your hands. The decisions you make during that time should favor your best shot at fatherhood. More interestingly, you don't have to wait for the third trimester to learn—your partner doesn't even need to first become pregnant for you to discover exciting ways to make first-time fatherhood a dream to live for. You can start now!

Chapter 1:

Becoming a Modern Dad

It takes a lot of effort to become today's dad, but once you establish the right foundation, the results will be worth it.

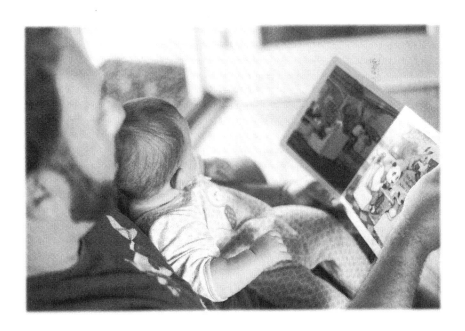

Emotional Planning and Preparation

If you just got the message, call, or took the test and just found out that your partner is pregnant, congratulations! Planned or not, you may feel different. As a first-time dad, you may find yourself experiencing all kinds of emotions from being excited to having anxiety, isolation, or probably feeling sad about it. Do not worry, it's normal to feel any of the aforementioned emotions. With that said, as you are about to enter this exciting journey of becoming a father or fatherhood, you will need to prepare yourself emotionally, physically, and mentally. It will not be a walk in the park but preparedness will make it easy for you to know what is coming in front of you. As you prepare for the beautiful addition in your life, you should welcome the idea that your way of living is about to change. It is also crucial for you to understand that your birthing partner will go through a lot of changes in the next nine months and the first year of your little one's existence.

Your new life as a dad will require you to learn how to take care of the baby and offer any help when your partner needs a hand. It is common for you to have increased stress as you attempt to strike a balance between assisting your spouse with the pregnancy and taking on more financial responsibility. When it gets overwhelming, do not be afraid to seek guidance from those who have walked through the road you are on and don't be afraid to go for counseling if you need it.

Developing your fatherly abilities will make it easier for you to see that you actually have this under control and are benefiting your family significantly. When you focus on the now and learn the right tricks and strategies, taking a step toward fatherhood will not always be hectic. You will soon come to cherish your newfound role in life.

Pregnancy Challenges

All good things do not come easily, the stress that pregnancy can impose on your relationship is real and you might be in a position where you are always conflicted. For instance, you might be concerned about the state of the economy or the health of your significant other. Your spouse may get concerned if you show less enthusiasm in the pregnancy than she does, or she may worry that she will become less beautiful as the pregnancy progresses because of the changes in her body. It's possible that the two of you have quite different perspectives on having sexual encounters while she is pregnant.

You and your partner may assist each other; feel encouraged and like you're working together by communicating with one another in an open and honest manner. Give one another time to talk and make an effort not to undermine the significance of the other person's emotions. There are moments when all you require is the sense that you are being heard and understood.

Physical Changes

Your partner's body undergoes many changes or modifications throughout pregnancy so she might need reassurance from time to time. After delivery, most of the changes disappear, but the new mom might not have enough patience to wait for her body to return to its pre-pregnancy state. Especially, where skin changes are the issue: Your partner might want to use beauty products for restoration. Although there is nothing wrong with a woman wanting some feminine confidence, some products might be unsafe for the baby. It is important that you both spend time to determine

which products are suitable for use and vice versa.

Most of the symptoms that result from hormonal changes during pregnancy are normal, but others might require medical attention.

Let's look at the normal physical changes you will see in your spouse.

- breast enlargement

Because hormones (estrogen mostly to be specific) are preparing the breasts for milk production, the breasts may increase in size. The number of milk-producing glands gradually rises and their capacity to create milk develops. Your partner will probably complain about her breasts being tender and hard. Her breasts will be more sensitive during this period.

- weight gain

It is possible that your partner will take a few extra pounds during pregnancy and this will be because of various factors which include organs like the uterus getting larger, your developing unborn getting bigger, and the placenta preparing itself for its new tasks. This weight gain will contribute to making her easily tired when she tries to do any physical activity. Your partner may also retain fluids and experience facial and limb edema (swelling). Blood and body fluids circulate more slowly because of this added weight and gravity, especially in the lower limbs.

- cervical changes

During pregnancy and childbirth, the cervix, which leads to the uterus, undergoes physical changes. The cervix's tissue thickens during pregnancy. The pressure of the developing baby may cause the cervix to relax and slightly enlarge up to a few weeks before giving birth.

- hair and nail changes

During pregnancy, you may see your birthing partner have changes in their hair and nail patterns. Hormonal changes may sometimes cause hair loss or excessive hair shedding.

- skin changes

You will notice a lot of skin changes in your partner as she is carrying your unborn child. One of those changes includes melasma, which is a blotchy, brownish tint that can affect the cheeks and forehead. The skin around your partner's nipples is also prone to darkening.

You will also notice a dark line at the center of your partner's abdomen. It is called the linea nigra and runs straight, along the umbilical area. This occurs when the placenta's hormone production drives the melanocytes to produce melanin. Melanocytes are the cells that make melanin, the dark brown skin pigment. Besides abdominal and facial skin changes, you may also notice the most well-known skin modification that is associated with pregnancy—striae gravidarum, commonly called stretch marks. They result from both physical stretching of the skin and the impact of hormone changes on the elasticity of the skin.

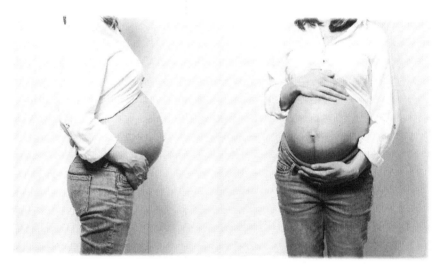

Physiological Changes

Your partner will not only have physical changes, but she will also have changes inside her body.

- body temperature

One of the first indications of pregnancy in your spouse is a rise in her basal body temperature. The mom-to-be will maintain a slightly greater core temperature throughout the pregnancy, and she will need to drink more water than her average intake. Without taking precautions to exercise properly and stay hydrated, she may be more susceptible to hyperthermia and dehydration.

- heart and blood vessels

Your woman's heart works harder during pregnancy because more blood needs to be pumped to the uterus as your unborn child develops. One-fifth of her blood supply is delivered to the uterus by the time pregnancy is over. The amount of blood the heart pumps rises by 30-50% during pregnancy. In addition, her blood vessels relax because of the pregnancy hormone progesterone, which reduces resistance and promotes blood flow. Also, her blood volume will increase up to 45% more than it was before she was pregnant.

- sensory changes

The visual, gustatory, and olfactory experiences that a woman has during pregnancy can be significantly altered.

- respiratory changes

When your partner is pregnant, there is an increase in the amount of oxygen her blood carries. Her blood arteries widen in order to meet the elevated demand for blood. This also increases the expectant mom's metabolic rate; therefore, she will need to consume more calories and exercise regularly.

Progesterone, a hormone that is continually created during pregnancy, tells the body to breathe more quickly and deeply. Because of this, a pregnant woman exhales more carbon dioxide to maintain a low level of gas.

Morning Sickness, Pregnancy Brain, and Cravings

Morning sickness is the popular name given to nausea and vomiting that pregnant women experience in the early stages of pregnancy. It is possible for your partner to have it and can often be experienced at any time of the day or night.

Signs and symptoms to help you identify morning sickness in the mom-to-be include: nausea and vomiting, which is often triggered by specific odors, certain kinds of foods, heat, and sometimes no triggers at all. Morning sickness is most common during the first trimester, symptoms in your spouse will improve when you both enter the second trimester.

There is a possibility of your partner having hyperemesis gravidarum, which is a severe form of morning sickness that occurs throughout pregnancy. This will be of great concern as your partner will be at high risk of being dehydrated and malnourished because she will not get enough fluids and nutrients from the water and food she will consume. She might require treatment from a professional, in a hospital.

Sex During Pregnancy

You probably have burning questions and one of them is will your sex life change while your partner is pregnant? Is it safe to have sex while pregnant? And when can you not engage in sexual activities during pregnancy?

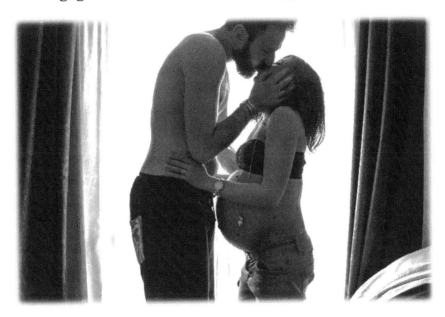

When your partner becomes pregnant, changes are inevitable in your sexual life. Her desire to have sexual encounters will either reduce or increase. The honest dialogue will be the key to a satisfying and safe sexual relationship during pregnancy; whether this means talking about how you feel, trying unique positions, or finding other ways to be intimate. This is because open communication is the key to a satisfying and safe sexual relationship during pregnancy.

You might be concerned that having sex will harm your unborn child. However, that should not cause you to worry because your unborn baby is safe in the amniotic sac. This means you will not harm the little one even if you engage in sexual activity. Therefore, as long as everything is going well with the pregnancy, it is okay to have sex and even orgasm while your partner is carrying the baby.

There are various scenarios in which having sex while pregnant could put the unborn child in danger. Those scenarios are if your partner has a history of cervical weakening, has symptoms suggesting that of a miscarriage or premature labor, has been suffering from significant cramping or pain in the abdomen region, or if she has placenta previa. You should not engage in sexual activities if your partner has been experiencing vaginal bleeding without a known cause. Seek medical help if you notice any of these.

Final Thoughts

Ancient times and traditions which did not require men to be part of the pregnancy and take care of the newborn are long behind us. Be a modern dad that will be on top of his game and be there for your unborn child and your partner because this is a time you will start bonding with your child. You are going to have challenges but just know you are not in it alone. And most importantly, don't forget to have fun as you gain new skills and knowledge on how you can assist your pregnant partner and your unborn. Remember, it gets easier with time.

Chapter 2:

Pregnancy Month by Month

This chapter is a guide to help you understand your little one's growth and some changes taking place in your partner's body during the course of the pregnancy.

The First Trimester

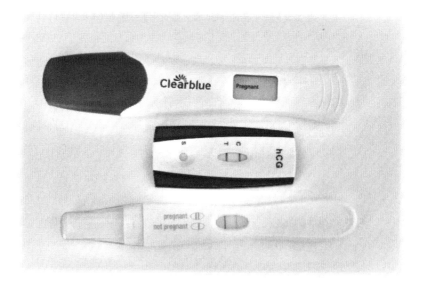

Month One

In preparation for pregnancy, the lining of your partner's uterus will become thicker. During the third week of her pregnancy, your partner may not experience any noticeable changes in her body. Even the famous sign, missed period, still hasn't happened at this point. However, your partner is close to missing her period because her hormones are sending signals to put menstruation on hold and focus on supporting the pregnancy. In its early days, the life growing in your partner's body does not resemble the looks of a baby yet because it is just a cluster of rapidly growing cells.

After the egg has been fertilized, a process called implantation takes place. This is when the ball of cells begins to attach itself onto your partner's uterine lining. The process may cause some light spotting. Apart from that, our partner may not notice any difference just yet, or her breasts may feel swollen and painful.

Month Two

In the second month, your partner's early signs of pregnancy may become more frequent. Your baby's umbilical cord forms to supply the growing life with oxygen and nutrients. When the second month begins, the amniotic sac and the placenta are still developing.

Your partner may put on some weight during this month, but if she is suffering from bad nausea, she might lose some pounds before it gets better. With fuller breasts and legs, your partner might report that her clothes feel tighter than before.

Your baby's ears begin to develop toward the end of the second month. With its webbed, tiny toes and fingers, the fetus can now enjoy unlimited swimming sessions in amniotic fluid. Because of the growing baby, your partner's heart pumps more blood to meet the increasing demand. She may experience mood swings during this month, so be careful not to poke her. Your doctor can now determine when your partner's due date will be.

Month Three

Your partner's uterus will continue to enlarge, and you may also notice her waistline becoming more prominent. Despite malleable bones, your unborn baby is beginning to take shape, but the bones are still malleable. Even though you are unable to feel the baby's movements at this point, you may be able to see them on an ultrasound.

Your partner will soon need maternity bras, so the last month of her first trimester may be the right time to start shopping for such items. Your baby's limbs become longer toward the end of this month, and they should be able to bend. Your baby's toes and fingers ditch the webbing and become distinct.

You may notice your partner's nails and hair growing and glowing during the third month of her pregnancy. However, some moms-to-be may also find that their skin is oily and prone to acne. Both the good and the unfavorable beauty changes are due to pregnancy hormones in your partner's body. By the end of the first trimester, your developing baby should have a distinct, baby-like profile.

The Second Trimester

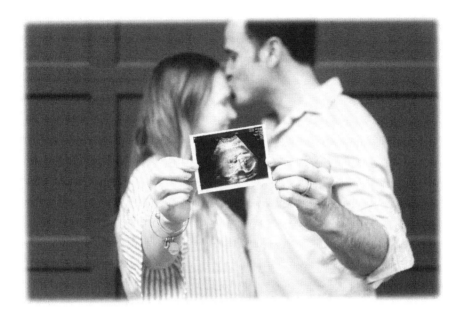

Month Four

Your partner's uterus has expanded quite a bit. It has reached the point where it is completely filling her pelvis and is beginning to grow into the abdomen. The round ball you feel when massaging your partner's belly is the baby's temporary home for the next few months. Although the baby's head is still a little too big, the other body parts are slowly catching up. Your little one's eyes are beginning to move into position. Your little one's backbone becomes flexible so the baby can move around more easily.

A few days into the second trimester, your partner's muscles and skin begin to stretch as they prepare to make room for the developing baby. The mom-to-be may also develop spider veins on her face and legs, but those will become less noticeable once the baby arrives. On the brighter side, your baby develops clear facial characteristics and distinct fingerprints are present. The baby's ears slowly move to their right position at the back of the head, the neck is getting longer, and the chin is becoming more prominent. Your little one starts to react to stimuli from the outside world. If you poke your partner's stomach, you will feel some movements as the baby tries to escape.

Your baby's eyebrows and the hair on top of its head have started to grow, and its bones are becoming denser. Your little one may have started sucking the thumbs when swimming gets tiring! In addition to the hair on your baby's head, they may now have fine, temporary hair covering them. The hair is known as lanugo and often sheds when the baby arrives. Although your baby's organs are completely formed, they continue to mature.

The baby's legs and arms start moving, and your partner may report quickening, a fluttering movement the unborn baby makes. Although their eyelids are still shut, your little one makes subtle eye movements too!

Month Five

Because of your partner's weight gain, her pregnancy is becoming more noticeable now. She might also have reported that her appetite has increased during this time. The baby's heart should be strong and pumping well by this time.

Your partner could experience an increase in pain in her lower back, and the pain might also extend to her navel and pubic area. Because the changes in circulation can cause her to feel dizzy, your partner should put getting up slowly into practice.

Your developing baby's reflexes are kicking in, and the baby is able to yawn, stretch, and even make faces. Because your little one's retinas are now responsive to light, the baby may move to protect the eyes if you shine a light on your partner's abdomen.

The bronchioles, which are the primary airways in your baby's lungs, begin to develop at this stage. Your baby's skin is still translucent and developing, so it vividly shows the blood vessels beneath it. The skin also develops a creamy-white protective layer known as vernix during this time.

Although her nausea and vomiting should have mostly subsided by this point, inflammation of your partner's mucous membranes can lead to symptoms such as stuffiness and nosebleeds. She might also develop some red marks on her face, arms, and shoulders due to dilatation of her blood vessels.

Because of the increased activity of your partner's thyroid gland, she may report that she sweats more than she did before the pregnancy. You may also notice that her breathing becomes more rapid, especially when she engages in physical activity.

Kegel exercises improve bladder control, so they can be very beneficial to your partner during this period. Your little one is now able to hear sounds such as the mother's voice when she talks or sings, her heartbeat, and even stomach sounds. This means you can bond with the baby by singing or talking to them when you are free as they also hear sounds from the outside world. By this time, you and your partner may see a lot of movement as your little one twists, wiggles, and turns.

Month Six

Later, during the second trimester, your partner may experience heartburn symptoms more frequently as her uterus puts more pressure on the stomach. She may also have dry or itchy skin, so you can help her stay comfortable by moisturizing it, especially her breasts, the abdomen, and the areas exposed to the air such as the face and hands. On a lighter note, your baby continues to grow and their muscles gain more strength with time.

Your little one may start having hiccups, which result in jerking movements. However, you can reassure your partner that the hiccups won't hurt the baby. As your partner's ligaments become loose in preparation for childbirth, she may complain about more pain in her back and around the hips. She might love to lie down and enjoy calming massages during this time, but don't be afraid to ask if she would like to try anything else too. Your partner might feel some mild cramping after having sexual intercourse, but a gentle massage should help ease her body. Your little one is beginning to produce white blood cells for assistance in warding off illness and infection in the future.

Around the end of the second trimester, you will notice the most rapid expansion of your partner's breasts, while the baby's skin gains an opaquer appearance rather than the transparent one.

The Third Trimester

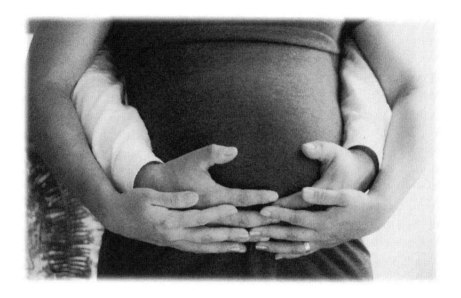

Month Seven

In the third trimester, your partner's uterus grows and expands above her belly button. She may complain about leg cramps, and shortness of breath, and her feet and ankles may have mild swelling. As the baby continues to grow bigger and stronger, your partner may also have Braxton Hicks contractions, a labor preparation sign that happens when her uterus is hardening and relaxing. With her abdomen looking all huge and the baby moving around in the womb, your partner may have difficulty falling and staying asleep.

As her uterus continues to press on other organs, your partner may complain about more discomfort, leg cramps, and clumsiness. You and your partner might want to start discussing the signs of preterm labor in order to be prepared if your little one ends up coming early. When labor is close, she may have lower back pain, abdominal cramps that feel similar to menstrual pain, and leaking amniotic fluid, among other signs. Your little one continues to kick and stretch, despite the uterine conditions being a little more limiting than before.

Your partner may feel more pain in her abdomen and pelvis later during the final trimester of the pregnancy as the baby is still pressing against her ribs. The baby's hair, eyelashes, and brows have grown well, and they look ready for the world. The tiny human in your partner's womb even makes red blood cells on their own! Your little one can now pick up certain sounds, such as music and voices they hear often. Your partner's stretch marks may appear more obvious, but it's almost time.

Month Eight

Your partner might notice a yellowish fluid leaking from her breasts. The fluid is called colostrum, and the body produces it in preparation for the common breast milk. As you enter the final weeks of the pregnancy, you may find that your partner's desire to have sexual encounters lessens, but if she is still up for it, having intercourse during this time won't hurt your little one.

The baby is exploring its newly found breathing ability and learning to blink. As your partner's uterus expands, she may prefer to eat more frequent but smaller meals to

28

avoid feeling uncomfortable. Your little one's brain can now send signals to regulate their body temperature.

Your partner's uterus is likely pressing firmly against her lower abdomen because her belly is expanded. This may also cause her rib cage and ribs to be in pain. In the third trimester, you may notice that your partner's navel is protruding or appears bigger, but don't be alarmed as that is another result of her expanding uterus. Your little one's skin now becomes pinkish rather than red. Apart from the lungs, which need a little more time, the baby's organs should be very close to being ready. The baby's fingernails have grown to cover the nail bed, but the toenails are yet to reach their full length.

Your growing little one continues to store fat beneath the skin in order to maintain their body temperature after birth. If you haven't already, the third trimester is the time for you and your partner to make sure you have enough baby clothes, furniture, and other equipment at least for the baby's first few weeks with you.

Month Nine

Over the course of the past few weeks, your partner's uterus has likely increased in size and moved closer to the top of her ribcage. It's also possible that her back will feel stiffer, and that she will have a heavy feeling in both her buttocks and her pelvis. Your little one is beginning to establish sleep patterns. The tiny human may move lower in the abdomen. If everything is going well, the baby should be moving into a head-down position to get ready for delivery.

Your partner is most likely experiencing a good deal of discomfort as the long-awaited day draws close. The baby's skin becomes smoother and less wrinkled, with its tiny legs getting rounder every day. It may be more difficult for the baby to move around as much as before, but they should still kick. Your little one's immune system uses antibodies from the mother to protect the baby from illness. The rate of the baby's growth slows down toward the end of the third trimester, but their fat cells continue to expand in preparation for the baby's new life with you.

By the end of the third trimester, your little one's skeleton is defined and the muscles are fully developed. The baby's lungs have reached their full potential and are now able to breathe outside the womb without difficulties. The baby's head should have descended into your partner's pelvis, and although it may cause her to experience feelings of fullness and discomfort, it is almost time! She may breathe easier when she lies on her back with her head lowered.

Your curious little one is now ready to join the family! They can now breathe, cry, and feed. However, if your partner's due date passes and the baby does not arrive, you don't have to stress about it because there's a way around it. Your partner might not want to consume any food during labor, but you should check with the healthcare team to see what food options are available.

Chapter 3:

Emotions and Support

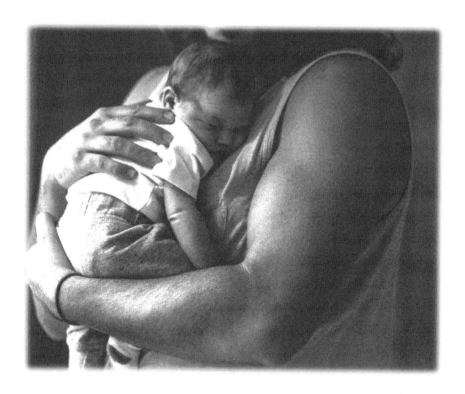

Preparing Your Mind to Become a Dad

Finding out that you will soon be a dad can bring up a range of feelings, including delight, surprise, and fear. When you are getting ready to become a father, it is critical that you give yourself plenty of time to prepare, seek advice from others, and carry out research on strategies to confront your fears.

You might not be the one who is carrying the baby in your body, but it does not imply that you are not a part of the experience of being pregnant or giving birth. Those who are considering adopting or using a surrogate can say the same thing; there are undoubtedly ways to feel connected in the process. There are a lot of books available on the market that are designed for future dads, but you don't have to restrict yourself to just reading those. You could also take part in some online communities that encourage dads to learn in a positive environment, free of judgment.

- Have conversations with your partner about parenting issues.

This time presents an excellent opportunity to engage in conversations about what kind of parent each of you intends to become. Are you both completely committed to breastfeeding the baby? Your support is very important to promote successful nursing. Do you want to put the baby to sleep in your room, in their cot, or in their own room? Are both of you planning to work soon after the baby arrives? What kind of preparations have you made for child care?

Keep in mind that both of you are only considering these ideas on a theoretical level for now. It's possible that your feelings will shift after your enchanting bundle of joy arrives. It's possible that breastfeeding will prove to be more difficult than you expected, or that you'll need to re-evaluate how you feel about using cloth diapers.

There are also conversations that won't be crucial just yet although they will be important in the future. Before your little one grows and starts acting out, you and your partner should have an open discussion about discipline, which should include strategies such as spanking and yelling. Is yelling at the child acceptable? When is it okay to give your little one a beating? Starting the conversation now will open those channels of communication and assist the two of you to get on the same page regarding parenting.

- Imagine the father you aspire to be.

It's easy to get into the trap of thinking that you'll never be able to live up to the standards set by the father you look up to or the dad character in the comedy show you enjoy watching the most. Spend some time assuring yourself that you will be an excellent father in your own special manner and then go about your day. Imagine what it would be like for you if that were to happen. What kinds of activities do you usually take part in? Where will you and your little one hang out when you are not at home? Which moments do you absolutely not want to miss at all costs?

If those suggestions aren't working, you can try visualizing your kid as an adult instead. What things do you hope people will say about you? Put your attention on the life lessons, the direction, and the love that you wish to pass on to the next generation. Consider your function in relation to that of your partner and think about how the two of you may complement one another. Researching the different approaches to parenting and figuring out which one agrees with you the most will help you decide the father you are going to be.

- Be a part of the process.

Take part fully in your partner's experience of carrying your little one. Spend some of your time engaging in pregnancy-related activities and maintain an active relationship with your partner. The first few days are critical because they determine how much you will be involved once your little one arrives. Every stage of development brings its own unique wonders and opportunities for extraordinary growth, and you don't want to miss any bit.

It would be great if you could attend all of your partner's doctor's appointments, but if you are always busy, you can at least try to attend the first one and the one where you get a chance to listen to the baby's heartbeat. Ask your doctor questions about the phases of pregnancy, the growth of your baby, and what changes are normal for your partner to experience. During your free time, you can also learn how to handle a newborn, discuss the various birthing alternatives and plans, and pack the hospital bag with your birthing partner. Have fun during the process and use it as an opportunity to strengthen the bond you share with your little one and the mom-to-be.

- Start working together as a team.

You and your birthing partner will benefit from thinking of yourselves as a team rather than just two individuals. Even if you do not have an ongoing romantic relationship with your baby's mom, you will always have a connection with your little one and that is worth co-operating with the mom-to-be. As you mentally prepare to become a father, it is best to avoid or give up the practice of keeping scores as if parenting is a game.

For instance, if your birthing partner is battling exhaustion and nausea, lending her a helping hand benefits both you and your little one. You can contribute to the shared goal of being there for your family in a variety of ways, such as providing food, improving your ability to housekeep, or just checking in on them regularly if you live apart.

- Figure out your finances.

The first few months of pregnancy are an excellent opportunity to analyze your financial situation. It is possible that the birthing partner may experience a loss of income, will be confronted with medical expenditures, and will be considering possibilities for paid or unpaid parental leave. Preparing both of you in advance for the financial situation can make the pregnancy live more peacefully.

Put your money in order, set up automated bill payments, pay any bills that are still outstanding, and try to be a few months ahead of yourself if you can. How? Debt consolidation or making active inquiries regarding employee benefits to help you are some examples of things that fall under this category. Because becoming a parent comes with a whole host of additional financial obligations, you should do everything in your power to make your current financial situation less stressful.

- Accept the possibility that your sexual life will change.

Becoming a dad will almost certainly have some kind of an impact on your sexual life. When you first find out that your partner is pregnant, you may have a wide range of feelings, including an incredible sense of connection to them and a desire for the intimacy of sex, anxiety about doing anything that might have an effect on the pregnancy, or simply a feeling of being puzzled. Another situation in which open communication is essential is this one.

You may look forward to hearing a lot of jokes mocking the fact that your sexual life is finished or making fun of the physical shifts that occur during pregnancy. These comments are not helpful as they disregard the emotional complexities that come with sexuality and parenthood. The truth is that returning to sexual activity after pregnancy will take some time, and we're not just talking about the recommended six-week period of rest and recuperation after giving birth and having a baby.

It is important to communicate with your partner about their needs and your own when it comes to matters of intimacy and sex. It is also crucial to be understanding when it comes to the changes you and the mom are going through, such as the inability to sleep and the emotional effect of being first-time parents. But sexual activity after giving birth can even be more satisfying. You are connected in ways that you have never been connected before, and the same experience of being parents can draw many couples even closer to one another.

- Create a budget for your household.

Consider the financial implications of being a parent with your significant other as you work on developing a spending plan for your family. The cost of everything from child care to breastfeeding experts to a crib that complies with safety standards should be overestimated. Even while all of these things fall within a certain price range, you should still make room in your budget for more expensive options so that splurging on expert support when you really need it won't ruin your financial situation. Whatever is left over can be put away in preparation for inevitable future expenses such as dental care, the cost of attending college or a trade school, the cost of family holidays, and more.

Bracing for Change

When you find out your partner is pregnant, you immediately realize that your life is about to change in so many ways. You might be curious about the degree to which your everyday life will change while she is carrying the baby. During the process, she will go through a lot of physical and emotional changes. Both large and minor shifts will take place. Some of these are to be anticipated, while others will take you by surprise.

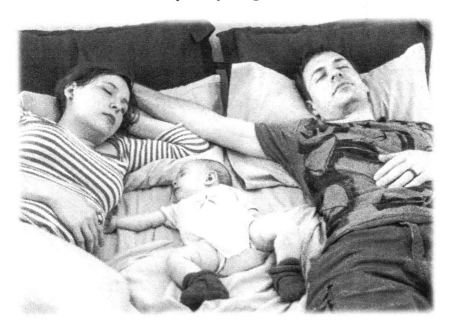

Your partner will have a greater need to use the restroom every now and then. You may start to notice that she has to use the restroom more frequently in the early stages of pregnancy, sometimes even before you are aware that she is carrying a bundle of life. This is completely normal and occurs as a result of her body having an increased amount of the pregnancy hormone called human chorionic gonadotropin (hCG). This hormone causes urination to become more frequent and may also be responsible for the disturbing morning sickness that's interfering with your partner's joy.

Your partner may put on more body weight as the baby develops. It is inevitable that your developing little one will add some of their own weight to the mom's, but still, your partner's body will also expand to make room for the innocent, new addition. Have a conversation with your physician about the healthy range for your partner's weight gain, and together stick to good eating habits as much as possible.

The mom-to-be will feel fatigued more frequently, and she may have a harder time falling or staying asleep. Because of the changes that are taking place in her body, you could discover that your partner gets weary more frequently. On the other hand, it may be more challenging for her to find a proper position in which to sleep, which may make it more difficult for her to have some rest in the first place. Sleeping on her side is your partner's safest and most comfortable posture during this time, but it can be difficult to adjust if she is used to sleeping on her tummy or back. You and your partner can talk to your prenatal care provider if she is having problems sleeping during her pregnancy.

As your partner's body changes, she may have trouble with nasal congestion. As if a blocked nasal passage is not enough, she may also experience frequent nosebleeds. This occurs as a result of her hormonal changes affecting her mucous membranes.

You and your partner will also have to adjust your schedules. You will need to put pregnancy-related appointments into consideration when making plans. This also means you may have to cancel some commitments to accommodate hospital appointments and other preparations for the baby.

Getting Involved

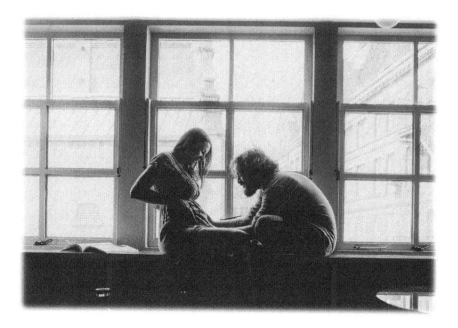

Pregnancy generally marks exciting times, but expecting parents may at times feel as though the process is loaded with a great deal of anxiety in addition to the joy that it comes with. You and your partner may have a lengthy list of things that you need to do before and when the baby arrives. The experience forces you to adapt to the shifting circumstances and unanswered questions regarding pregnancy and childbirth.

On the brighter side, the experience may strengthen your bond with the expectant mom and boost your chances of working together as a team because pregnancy forces you to show support for one another.

It is important that you educate yourself on how to embrace pregnancy changes with your partner especially because this will be your first little one.

When supporting your partner, you can try to:

- take her to prenatal appointments
- help her when making choices about prenatal tests
- attend childbirth classes with her

Your partner needs encouragement and reassurance from you, so you can help by staying close and asking her what you can help with. Given all the changes taking place in her body, the hormones can be quite confusing, so your partner needs to feel your affection to know you are still with her. You can provide emotional support by holding hands and giving her warm embraces.

- Attempt to consume as much nutritious foods as you can because this will assist her in eating healthily.
- Assist her in making necessary adjustments to her way of life. Because she can't consume alcohol and may reduce her caffeine intake, you can decide to give up drinking alcohol and coffee entirely or cut back significantly. If you have been contemplating some adjustments to your way of life, now might be a suitable moment to put those plans into action.
- Encourage your partner to rest often and take naps during the day if necessary. This is because her pregnancy hormones may cause changes in her activity level and her desire for sleep.

- You can also go on walks with your partner. This gives you both a chance to exercise as well as an opportunity to chat with other people.

Some women may wish to have less sexual activity when they are pregnant. As the baby continues to grow, your partner could experience feelings of exhaustion and discomfort. She could also feel insecure because of the changes occurring in her body. However, there are other pregnant women who crave more sex when they are pregnant. It is important to have a conversation with your partner about her feelings regarding pregnancy sex. Encourage her to be open so you can make informed adjustments to your intimate relationship.

As for physical support, get used to taking care of your home whenever you are free. This is of utmost importance during those times when the mom-to-be is feeling very exhausted, as well as in situations where certain odors from the kitchen cause her to feel queasy.

If you are a smoker, you might want to avoid doing so in her presence. Should you feel you want to quit, you can even enroll in a program to help you stop smoking altogether. If you don't intend to stop, you can try to reduce the number of cigarettes you consume each day, or simply step out from home.

As the pregnancy progresses, your partner might also appreciate getting relaxing massages on her back to help relieve some of the aches and stress that come with pregnancy.

It is important to note, dear dad-to-be, that this does not mean everyone is counting on you to do and give everything during pregnancy. Even if the surrounding people may focus more on your partner and the unborn baby, it does not mean that your family and friends have forgotten about you.

Have a lot of in-depth conversations with the mom-to-be about how the two of you feel. In the same way your partner opens up to you about her needs, you can do the same about yours without anyone thinking you are being weak, lazy, or neglectful. For instance, if your work schedule is tight and you want to rest on the day she wants to attend a hospital appointment, you can just let her know. Chances are your partner will appreciate that you were honest with her instead of forcing yourself to escort her, only to doze off in the waiting room.

Discuss with your partner what role you would like to have during labor and childbirth. Some expecting mothers want their partners to be in the room when their baby arrives, but others do not. Apart from that, other dads-to-be may experience anxiety and decide they would rather not be there. You and your birthing partner should both be able to work together and determine what is in your best interests.

You can also make contact with the other dads, including those who are expecting, to discuss experiences, ideas, and recommendations. Attending childbirth classes may provide you with the opportunity to network with other men in your situation.

Announcing the News

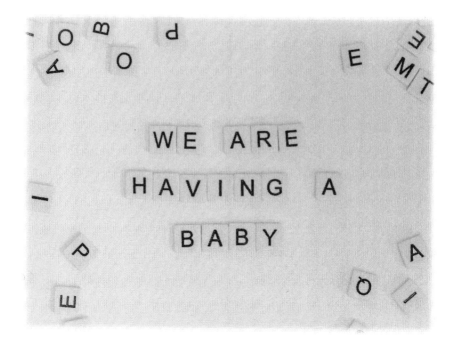

Making an announcement about pregnancy is a big deal because expecting a baby is a special kind of news. When you and your partner find out you are pregnant, you may feel as though you have won a lottery, especially if you have been trying for a baby. You may want to tell everyone, but you have to be cautious about when and how you break the news. So, when is the appropriate time to share the news that you are expecting? The timing sorely relies on what you and your partner decide.

Most couples may choose to announce their pregnancy after the 14-week mark; however, others choose to wait until after four to five months. They often do this to find out the baby's gender and ensure that the ultrasound results are normal before celebrating with others. However, you do not need to know the gender of the baby in order to announce that you are expecting. If you find abnormal ultrasound results after having shared the news already, you may appreciate the external support from friends and family.

You might decide to break the news to your immediate family and a few close friends before you break it to the rest of the world, or you might choose to tell everyone at the same time.

If you are not prepared to reveal the information, do not do so. When people you know notice that your partner hasn't been drinking her wine, they may try to coax the information out of you in order to satisfy their curiosity. However, do not feel obligated to reveal anything if you are both not yet prepared to do so. If you find yourselves in such a situation, you can simply change the subject or tell the curious person that you can only be sure when it shows.

Once you and your partner are ready, you should first share it with those who are closest to you. It will make the soon-to-be grandparents feel unimportant if they see it posted on Instagram before you call them with the good news. They should not find out together with the general public when it doesn't hurt to give them a call if they are far away.

Always be mindful of who you are sharing your news with. If you publicly post pictures of your developing fetus on Facebook or leave the post open to friends of friends, you might want to remind yourselves that you can no longer control what other people use the pictures for. This simply means if you are going to celebrate with a big audience, you may not afford to be as casual and free as you can be when sharing with close friends and family.

Chapter 4:

Birth Logistics

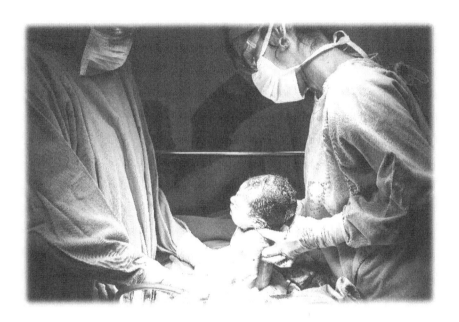

Choosing Your Hospital

How would you like your partner's labor and delivery process to go if you could have whatever you want? Bear in mind that it is possible for her to end up with a different obstetrician based on the on-call schedule that the doctors follow. If your partner goes into labor at night, she could end up having any obstetrician gynecologist who is working that shift, but even if it's during the day, it is also possible for her to deliver with the help of someone you have never discussed anything with before. Such situations make it crucial to look around for hospitals you are most comfortable with before the baby arrives. Finding the right maternity hospital has a significant impact on how your partner feels about the birthing experience, regardless of how things turn out during the process.

- Start with the fundamentals.

You and your partner might not be able to just start off anywhere for labor and delivery because of the high medical and travel expenses, as well as the restrictions placed on health insurance covers. Your insurance provider decides which hospitals and doctors it covers, so, they choose which maternity care facilities your partner can use. Your options may be limited further by other aspects, such as the location in which you reside, and the state of your partner's health in general.

- Prepare.

Because you will want to do little more than rest and take care of your new baby when you get back home, it is important that you and your partner make as many preparations as you can in advance.

If you have the means to do so, you should stock up on necessities such as toilet paper, maternity pads, and diapers well ahead of your partner's pregnancy clock. You and your partner can even prepare meals in advance and put them in your freezer for after the baby arrives because there will be plenty of things to do then.

When choosing a hospital, you will want to study and discuss some of the following factors:

- Provision for insurance coverage.

It is important to find maternity hospitals where doctors accept your insurance, given the wide range of possibilities for coverage both outside and within your insurance network.

- The amount of time it takes to the target hospital from your house.

You may not want to pick a hospital that is very far away or one that is difficult to reach due to a poor road network. This is because you don't have to worry about traffic congestion when your little one is already on the way. If the distance between your place of residence and the hospital interferes with the childbirth outcome, that defeats the entire purpose of choosing a maternity hospital. In such instances, you would realize you would have done well to choose a nearby hospital.

- Locations that can accommodate high-risk pregnancies.

If your partner has had a high-risk pregnancy or she has pre-existing health problems that may interfere with her pregnancy, the maternity hospital of your choice should be able to handle the worst-case scenario. Examples of factors you would want to consider include the availability of a blood bank, a neonatal intensive care unit (NICU), their ability to monitor your partner should she need to induce labor, and many more. High-risk pregnancies require proper medical care, so this is very critical if there are any chances your situation could become complicated.

Strategies for Selecting a Maternity Hospital

There is no such thing as picking a birthplace too early. The majority of women start seriously searching for the birthplace of their choice after they have positive test results for pregnancy, but some may consider where to deliver from even before they become pregnant, and that is also fine. Although you and your partner are free to change doctors at any time during the pregnancy, it is in your best interest to find a health-care provider you are comfortable with while you still have plenty of time.

- Consider your delivery options.

Discuss how your partner likes the labor and delivery to go and also let her know if you have any special requests or wishes. Use this chance to also talk about other important things related to the labor and delivery process. There are differences in the degree to which certain maternity hospitals encourage mom-to-be to give birth naturally. Some places have rules that restrict the number of people who can visit, but you will also have to consider that. To have a memorable experience, determine what makes you and your partner the most at ease. You can carry out some research and find out the following things in order to prevent any unpleasant surprises from occurring:

○ Where can we get the hospital guidelines?

Some hospitals have rules that limit the number of personal support people who can be in the room with the expecting mom while she is giving birth. You would do well to ask who they permit to enter if your partner values the presence of other family members or friends. While some countries require that pregnant women remain connected to a device that monitors the fetus's heart for the entirety of the labor process, others permit expecting moms to just be monitored at time intervals. If your partner is nervous, she could appreciate being monitored throughout the process, but if she is calm, being hooked up to the fetal heart monitor can be uncomfortable.

○ Do the hospital's guidelines resonate with what you and your partner want?

You may want to know if the hospital of your choice has special areas for various forms of natural childbirth, such as water birth. You can also ask if the hospital you want to pick has lactation consultants to assist with nursing once the baby arrives because the baby might not suck well without first getting the hang of it. It is important to find out about pain-management options the hospital offers. Does it support moms who want epidurals, as well as those who do not? If your partner receives an epidural to deal with the pain of childbirth, she will need an anesthesiologist to monitor her throughout.

     ○ If the obstetrician is unavailable when it's time for delivery, what are the next steps?

It is crucial that you and your partner know if the hospital has a plan in case of an emergency. A backup system is helpful whether the crisis is because your partner's initial doctor is not working at that time or because the mom-to-be needs a higher level of care.

     ○ What kind of amenities are included in the room?

It is worth exploring whether your partner wants to give birth at a maternity hospital that offers private rooms after delivery or if she is fine being in a shared room with another new mom. If your partner is in a private postpartum room, you and the baby could be there with her if the baby does not have problems that require special care. In a shared room, however, you may not be able to spend time with your partner as the other occupant would need her privacy. Sometimes, babies are moved to a nursery in the hospital, so you might also want to ask if it is possible for your little one to remain in the same room as the mother.

You and your partner might be able to get vital information about your target hospitals through online reviews and other evaluations, but you can also ask friends or family members who gave birth at the hospitals. You can try to talk to a large number of friends, family members, and even workmates about their childbirth experiences at different hospitals on your list of potential birthplaces. Your partner can also talk to the mothers in her life to get their thoughts on your list of potential hospitals. If you don't have friends who have had this experience, she can browse around the internet or join some groups for future parents.

Your Hospital Bag

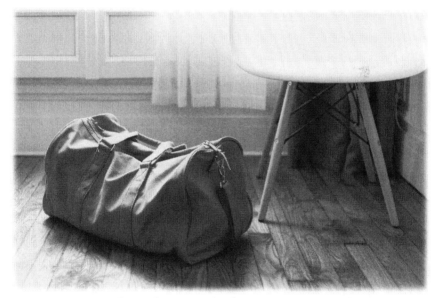

First, you need to figure out how to get to the hospital when the time comes. Because you may need to visit the hospital even during odd hours, you should make the preparations ahead of time. If you intend to use your car, be sure it's working well and has enough fuel to get to the hospital and back. Even so, you need a backup plan, so you ask a friend for help, or perhaps you can set transport money aside in advance.

For your partner, you may need:

- any special medicines she may be taking
- her hospital notes and birth plan
- breast pads
- loose, comfortable clothes to wear while waiting for the baby to arrive
- slippers for the bathroom
- a few supportive bras and nursing bras if she will breastfeed
- packed toiletry bag
- 2 packets of maternity pads
- loose-fitting nightwear
- item to help her relax while waiting for the baby
- approved snacks and drinks
- towels

For your little one, you may need:

- a car seat
- vests and bodysuits
- a clean baby blanket
- booties, mittens, and hats
- feeding bibs
- a full outfit for the trip home
- nappies or diaper

Prenatal Visits and Exams

It is very crucial that your partner attends all their prenatal appointments. You can show support by going with her, but if that does not favor your schedule, you may still find other ways to be involved. The mom-to-be should have all her exams on time to avoid complications and so her healthcare providers can catch any abnormalities early.

Baby Gender

Whether you and your partner choose to know your little one's sex in advance or you feel it's better to wait for the big day to be a surprise, no one can force you to decide otherwise. However, both options have their own advantages and disadvantages.

The advantages of knowing include:

- more time to adjust to reality if you or your partner wanted different sex for the baby
- informed preparation
- fun bonding time and parties that are in line with the baby's gender
- curiosity satisfaction
- enough time to choose the right name

The disadvantages of knowing include:

- the test could be wrong.
- too many gender-specific baby wear
- no surprises

The advantages of not knowing include:

- surprise joy
- fun choosing both male and female names
- No need to deal with disappointed family members who were hoping for a different gender during pregnancy

The disadvantages of not knowing include:

- The curiosity can drive you and your partner crazy
- Family and friends will pester you to find out
- less room for personalization

Choosing a Name

When you find out you're going to be a parent, you might already have a lengthy list of potential baby names compiled, broken down into categories such as girl names, boy names, and gender-neutral names. However, not everyone does this.

The decision of what name to give your child is important and you will need to make it with your partner. Although it has the potential to be enjoyable, the weight of duty that comes with naming your tiny human may make it feel quite scary. Here are some pointers that can help you determine whether or not the ideal name is the right name:

- put the initials in written form
- make sure there are no legal issues with the name
- think about the names you will give your baby's future siblings
- check for alternate spellings
- take care not to confuse the meanings
- search if there are other names that are too similar
- consider the uniqueness of each option
- consider other external elements

Chapter 5:

The Birth

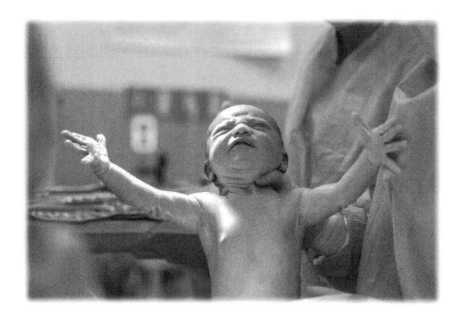

Is Your Partner Having Contractions?

To understand contractions and how they come about you need to know that the uterine muscle, which is the strongest muscle in a woman's body, goes through recurrent bouts of contracting and relaxing as part of the labor process. Oxytocin is a hormone that is released by the pituitary gland in response to a stimulus that causes the uterine muscle to contract tightly. It is impossible to determine exactly when the contractions of actual labor will begin though you can expect your partner to have them when they are at term.

Pregnant women often describe contractions as a cramping or tightening sensation that begins from the back and sweeps around to the front in a wave-like manner. Your spouse will complain of abdominal pain which will be regular, sustained, and will become stronger with time. Some women have described contractions as a sensation of pressure on the back. When a contraction is taking place, the abdomen will feel very firm when touched. The labor process occurs before giving birth and is accompanied by a sequence of contractions. These contractions force the upper area of the uterus, known as the fundus, to constrict and thicken, whereas the lower portion of the uterus and the cervix expand and relax. This allows the baby to move from the top part of the uterus into the birth canal so that it may come out properly.

Do You Know the Difference Between False and Real Labor?

The contractions that were described above are associated with real labor but do you know that there are also False contractions? and the next question is how would you differentiate if your partner is having real labor contractions or false labor contractions?

Let's get to it.

In the last few weeks of pregnancy, your partner might

experience some contractions. However, these contractions may not necessarily indicate the beginning of labor: this is called false labor. Braxton Hicks contractions, often known as false labor, is the medical term for these cramps.

Braxton Hicks contractions are unpredictable. They do not occur in closer proximity to one another compared to true labor contractions. When your partner moves around, changes positions, or rests, she will frequently get relief from them. Real labor contractions have a pattern of being regular, happening in closer proximity, getting stronger, and continuing even when your laboring partner changes position, rests or moves about.

Timing the duration of her contractions can help you differentiate between true labor and fake labor.

Consider the amount of time that elapses between the beginning of one contraction and the beginning of the next contraction, and take into account the gap in time between them as well. Make an appointment to see your obstetrician as soon as possible if any of the following apply to her contractions:

- She is experiencing consistent and severe pain.
- they last least thirty to sixty seconds
- She doesn't have relief even when she lies down.
- they occur at regular intervals, typically 5–10 minutes
- Vaginal bleeding accompanies the contractions.

Did Her Water Break?

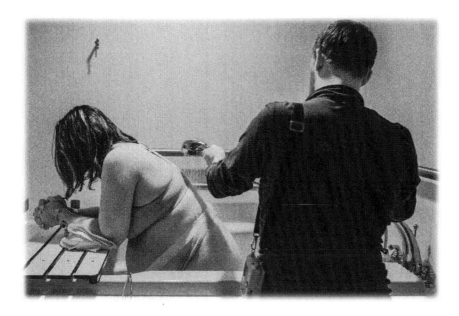

Before talking about the water breaking, you have to know where the water comes from. In the amniotic sac, the amniotic fluid that fills the amniotic sac cushions and protects your unborn child during your partner's pregnancy. In addition to assisting in the development of your baby's lungs and renal system, amniotic fluid also maintains a constant temperature in the surrounding area. Although the urine of your unborn child makes up the majority of the fluid in the second trimester of pregnancy, there are also nutrients, hormones, and antibodies (which help the body fight infection) present in this fluid. The sac's membranes can rupture before the beginning of labor, later on during labor, or even before labor begins in certain situations. This can happen at any point. This phenomenon is referred to as water breaking.

It is frequently one of the earliest signals that labor is about to begin.

It might be difficult for your spouse to be certain that she will recognize when her water has broken and there are a variety of experiences that other women have had when their waters broke in the late stages of pregnancy. The following are the most reliable indications that can give you a clue that your partner's water has broken:

- The mom-to-be has no control over the amount of fluid leaking.

When her water finally breaks, she can experience a torrent of amniotic fluid pouring out of her body, or she might simply notice a sluggish drip. The amount depends on where exactly the rapture has taken place; if the amniotic sac ruptures below the baby's head, then fluid will accumulate and will pour out in larger quantities. However, if the membrane rupture occurs higher in the womb, the fluid will have to trickle down between the sac and the uterine lining, which will cause a flow that is not as heavy.

- She might experience a urinating sensation

During the third trimester of pregnancy, some women experience urinary incontinence, which may feel similar to the onset of water breaking. If your spouse says she just lost control and she thinks she has passed urine but you can't tell the difference between water breaking and urine, then this is how you can identify the difference between them: Urine has a yellowish hue and smells like ammonia, but amniotic fluid is typically odorless. Urine also has a different consistency. Amniotic fluid is typically odorless; nevertheless, some individuals report smelling an unpleasant aroma similar to that of semen or chlorine. Additionally, it may be transparent or have a faint pink hue with red streaks running through it.

- It is light and not sticky, like other discharges.

You and your spouse are more likely to confuse the rupturing of membranes with other discharge, particularly if the discharge is coming out slowly. In most cases, amniotic fluid, unlike other vaginal discharge, does not have a discernible odor; Some discharges like leukorrhea are more viscous and may have the appearance of clear or milky white mucus. Amniotic fluid is usually of a very runny consistency.

You should be aware that if her water breaks before term without signs of labor such as contractions, that is called the preterm premature rupture of membranes (PPROM). If your partner experiences this emergency situation, you should immediately seek medical attention because it comes with an increased risk of infection. The mom-to-be will most likely be delivered when taken to the hospital because the baby is now at term.

What If She Needs an Emergency Birth at Home?

Do you fear that your partner might go into labor while at home and be unable to go to a hospital?

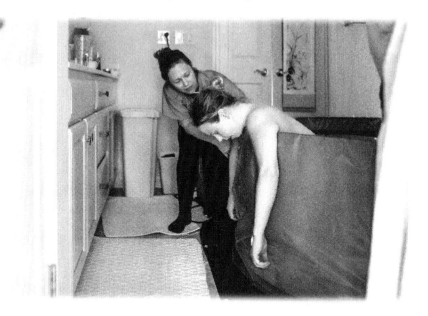

Unlike the dramatic movies that show this happening, in real life, the probability of this occurring to you and your partner is extremely low because signs of labor will manifest themselves hours before childbirth. Another reason is that labor progresses slowly in first-time mothers, although it is quicker in mothers who have given birth before.

If you find yourself in this position, do not worry, here are some steps to guide you:

- Evaluate the situation.

Before everything else, how do you tell if the baby is coming soon and you won't make it to the hospital? Even though each woman's labor is unique, if she is complaining of feeling strong, protracted, regular contractions that are normally spaced no more than five minutes apart, or if her water has burst and she feels a strong urge to push, she is showing indicators that delivery is about to happen.

- Call the emergency line.

Call 911. Inform the dispatcher that you are expecting a baby and that you require an emergency medical team right away.

- Do not lock your doors and call for help.

Keep your door unlocked so the emergency personnel may enter when they arrive. Later, you might not be able to reach the door. Call a friend or neighbor if other family members are not home.

- Call your midwife or physician.

Up until help arrives, they will stay on the phone to help and guide you.

- Get the necessities.

Grab some blankets, sheets, or towels. So that you may immediately cover your partner and your newborn after giving delivery, place one underneath her and have the others close by.

- Undress her or help her into a clean gown.

Remove her clothing and underwear. Help her lay down or raise the seat. If she gives birth while standing, your baby can fall and sustain catastrophic injuries.

- Be calm.

Be as calm as you can. Deliveries are often simple for babies who arrive quickly. Try to hold back the temptation to shove. Encourage her to be patient and encourage breathing exercises.

Here is how you proceed:

As carefully as you can, when the head is outside, assist your baby outside. If your baby's umbilical cord is around their neck, either gently ease it over their head or make a loop so the rest of their body may pass through it. Place your newborn on the mother's belly or chest so that skin-to-skin contact can keep him warm and comforted. Then, wrap him in a fresh towel. Wipe your baby's mouth and nose; if you have a penguin's sucker use it to remove extra fluid from your baby's mouth and nostrils to encourage initial breaths and aid in amniotic fluid drainage. The newborn begins breathing once they cry.

- Avoid cutting or tying the umbilical cord.

It may be challenging to cut the cord by oneself in a clean manner; yet, doing so could put your baby at risk for infection. In addition, roughly 30% of your baby's blood is still in the placenta at the moment of birth, which can provide them with two to five minutes of oxygen which can be lifesaving if they haven't begun breathing on their own, and professional help hasn't arrived yet.

- Encourage breastfeeding.

Encourage your spouse to breastfeed your baby while you wait for medical assistance, but only if you can maintain the umbilical cord loose rather than taut. Sometimes, if the placenta is still inside her, the cord won't be long enough for you to bring your infant to the mother's breast. In addition to providing comfort and security, the act of your baby sucking will cause your partner's body to create more oxytocin. This hormone induces contractions and aids in the delivery of the placenta.

- Deliver the placenta.

Although it will likely be far less intense than what she experienced during labor and delivery, she will probably experience pelvic pressure and contractions. The placenta may come out spontaneously or not. To deliver the placenta, avoid pulling on the cord. The placenta can stay in your uterus until aid arrives if necessary.

Chapter 6:

What Happens Next?

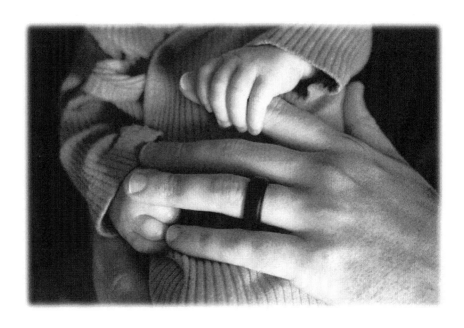

Right After Birth

Your partner's healthcare team will lift the baby up to her for skin-to-skin contact right after birth. This is important as it provides the baby with warmth in the outside environment. Apart from warmth, it also promotes bonding between the mother and the baby. Your baby's medical team will dry and then wrap the tiny human in a towel to prevent the baby from becoming chilly either before or immediately after they clamp the cord. While doing this, your partner can still hold the baby close.

Some new babies require a little assistance to help with their breathing, and your little one's nose and mouth may need to be cleaned of mucus. Depending on the situation, your baby might be moved to a different area of the delivery room for some oxygen, then the medical team will return your little one as soon as possible.

The medical team will examine, weigh, and measure your new bundle of happiness. After that, they will give the baby a wristband or anklet for identification. Your little one will also receive vitamin K to lessen the risk of a rare bleeding condition known as infant hemorrhagic illness. If you prefer that the baby gets it orally, they will require more doses than they would with an injection.

If your partner gets small tears and grazes during childbirth, they may not require sutures because they often heal on their own, but if she has major tears or had an episiotomy, she will need stitches. If nothing is wrong with the baby, your partner can even rock the baby while her doctor works. If she had an epidural, her anesthesiologist may need to top it up, and if she hadn't, the doctor may suggest a local anesthetic to numb the area.

After everything is done and your partner has to move to the postnatal ward, her midwife or other nurses will assist her in getting clean and dressed.

The First Bath

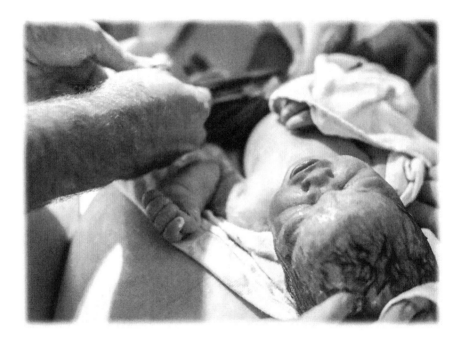

If you have questions about when it is appropriate to give your newborn baby a bath, you have complete control over the timing. The key element is that you choose a time when you won't be disturbed or tempted to rush through the process because your little one will be very fragile in the first few months. Some parents follow their tradition when bathing their babies for the first time, but it is best that you give your new joy their first bath within a week of their birth.

Try to avoid bathing your little one when they are overtired or immediately after feeding them. If your baby just refueled, you will want to wait a little bit so their meal can settle. Bathing your newborn when they are too tired or sleepy is a bad idea for a variety of reasons, but even you wouldn't want someone interrupting your deep sleep so you can bathe.

Some people prefer to bathe their babies in the morning because the little ones are often more alert at that time, but others prefer early evenings as part of winding down for the day. You can incorporate a soothing bedtime routine for your little one when it is time to rest in the evening.

It is important to keep in mind, however, that newborns do not require a lot of bathing, and at first, you will just be giving your little one a quick sponge bath until their umbilical cord stump falls off, which often occurs anywhere from one to three weeks after birth.

Choosing a Pediatrician

If you approach people you know and trust, including friends and family, for guidance in this area, you won't make a mistake since you'll get an honest response and a valuable recommendation from at least one person.

Do your homework, check their credentials, think about how easily you can get in touch with them, and make sure you're comfortable working with them.

Exams and Tests

Checking newborns after birth helps to identify critical health issues. Newborn screening is performed on every single baby, but these mandatory examinations are determined on a state-by-state basis. In most instances, the screening tests return normal results, but if they are abnormal, the baby will have a diagnostic test to determine what is wrong.

The majority of the time, medical issues that are detected early through screening of newborns can be cured. Treatment at an early stage is essential because it has the potential to help prevent more significant health issues for your little one.

- Blood test

The majority of newborn screenings include taking a blood sample to look for unusual but potentially life-threatening diseases. To perform a blood test, a medical professional will prick your little one and collect a few droplets of blood. They will then deliver the blood sample to a laboratory for analysis. The blood test results are usually ready from a few hours to about five days, but whether they are early or late depends on the hospital and laboratory involved. You and your partner can ask the medical personnel taking care of your little one if you want to find out more about when the results will be ready.

- Hearing screening

This test will be able to detect if your baby has issues with hearing. In order to do this test, your healthcare practitioner will insert very small earphones into your little one's ears and then use specialized computers to evaluate the baby's reaction to sound.

- Cardiac examination

The purpose of this test is to screen new babies for the category of cardiac disorders known as critical congenital heart defects (CHDs). The test involves a straightforward procedure known as pulse oximetry which measures the amount of oxygen in your baby's blood.

If the findings from these tests are also abnormal, your healthcare professional will be able to advise you on the next steps to take for your little one.

Setting Limits

If you and your partner are going to receive help when taking care of the baby, you will notice differences in the way other people handle babies. Some of the methods are correct but different from yours. However, other strategies which people use are wrong and can be dangerous, so you will need to set boundaries and educate those helping you.

Inform your loved ones, including your friends and family, on the appropriate way to hold and interact with the infant. Be careful not to offend the people supporting you, especially the elderly who may be resistant to your modern-dad strategies.

Prepare yourself for people to judge and make you feel uncomfortable. Being a dad is fun, so if you face resistance or harsh judgment, just focus your mind on being the best dad your little joy can have.

Chapter 7:

Sudden Infant Death Syndrome

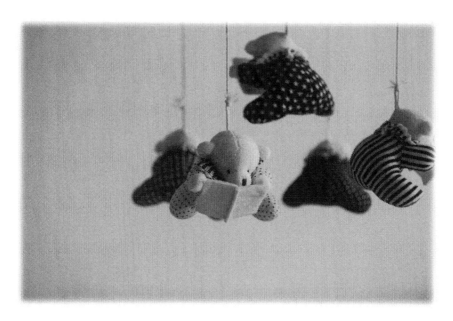

The phrase *sudden infant death syndrome* (SIDS) refers to the sudden or unexpected death of an infant. An infant is a baby that is less than one-year-old. These fatalities frequently occur while the baby is sleeping or in a sleeping space, they can happen in a baby who is healthy and has had no underlying problem. Because newborns frequently pass away in their cribs, SIDS is also referred to as crib death.

If you are wondering what causes sudden infant death, you are not alone. An infant's risk of SIDS may increase because of a confluence of physical and sleep-related environmental variables. This means the state of their health, sleep positions, and what's around them can contribute to them being a victim of sudden infant death syndrome. Risk factors differ from one baby to another.

Although they are unsure, medical officers have some theories and suggestions as to why this happens. Some newborns have a gene or a genetic mutation that results in specific health issues that can cause SIDS. Let us discuss other reasons below:

- Sometimes SIDS can happen if there is a hidden health issue, such as brain abnormalities in the infant.
  - A portion of the brain that regulates respiration, heart rate, blood pressure, temperature, and waking from sleep is affected in some newborns. This can lead to them having SIDS due to them not having an autonomic function in these activities.
- Low birth weight.
  - A newborn's brain may not have fully developed if he or she is born prematurely, in which case the baby will likely have less control over natural functions like breathing and pumping of blood by the heart. In addition, babies that are born with low birth weight are at an increased risk of having infections and poor temperature control.
- Passive smoking.
  - Secondhand smoking can cause harm to the baby as it can impair the baby's breathing and heart function. In addition, a

respiratory illness can also be a contributing factor to having SIDS.

- Making the baby sleep on one side or their abdomen.
  - Babies put to sleep in these positions are at greater risk of having breathing issues than babies put to sleep on their backs. Breathing issues include the possibility of the baby breathing in his or her own air which he or she has been breathing out which will lead to carbon dioxide build-up in the baby's body leading to respiratory compromise.
- Making your baby sleep on a soft mattress.
  - As you start your journey of being a new father, you might think that getting a soft mattress for your newborn is a good idea because you want them to be comfortable but an infant's airway might become blocked if they are lying face down on a soft mattress, waterbed, or fluffy blanket which will lead to SIDS.
- Sharing a bed with the baby.
  - As a new parent, you might think sharing a bed with your newborn is good for you and the new mom because of easy accessibility when it's time to assist the baby with what they need, but sharing a bed with your little one increases their risk of SIDS. While an infant's risk of SIDS reduces if they sleep in the same room as you, that risk rises if they share a bed with you or other people.

- Overheating.
  - A baby's risk of SIDS can increase if they are excessively warm while sleeping.

Keep in mind that none of these alone suffices to cause SIDS.

So, what are the risk factors?

- Family history.
  - There is an increased risk for a baby if an older sibling or cousin has died from sudden infant death syndrome (SIDS).
- Age
  - The period between the first to the fourth months of a baby's life is when they are at their most susceptible to being victims of SIDS.
- Sex
  - Boys have a little higher risk of passing away from SIDS than girls do.
- Race
  - African-Americans, Native Americans, and Alaska Natives are the demographic in whom statistics show this phenomenon most often. The reasons it affects these demographics are unknown.
- Premature birth
  - Full-term infants (those that completed 39 weeks of pregnancy) or term babies (37 to 40 weeks) are less likely to be affected by it compared to premature infants, especially those who are born very small.

Other risk factors are directly related to the condition of the parents. There is an increased risk of this happening to a child whose mother:

- gets little to no prenatal care
- is younger than 20 years of age
- smokes, uses illegal drugs, or consumes alcohol

Another factor that may raise the risk of a baby having SIDS is if the father does drugs, abuses alcohol, or smokes around the baby.

Guidelines From Pediatricians

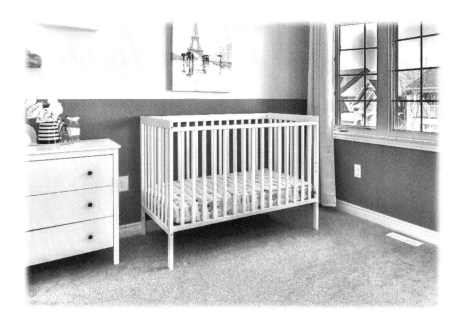

There is no failsafe technique for preventing sudden infant death syndrome (SIDS), but you can make the sleeping environment safer for your baby by adhering to the following suggestions, which experienced pediatricians recommend:

- Place the little one to sleep on their back for every sleep.

The supine posture is the one that you should use for your baby's sleep from the time they are born until they reach the age of one. You and your partner should do this at all times. Not only do experts discourage that your little one sleeps on their side, the position is also dangerous. It is vital that you position your newborn baby to sleep in the supine position as soon as it is possible because they have a higher risk of developing sudden infant death syndrome. You, your partner, and any other caregivers should do this every time the baby goes to sleep. It is okay for your baby to lie in either the prone or the lateral position as long as they are awake and you are there to monitor them. The prone position allows your little one to lie on their abdomen while the lateral position allows them to lie on their side.

- Use a sleeping aid surface that is dense.

When you ensure your infant sleeps on a flat, firm surface (such as a mattress in a safety-approved crib) with only a fitted sheet and no other bedding or soft items, you reduce the baby's risk of suffocating or developing sudden infant death syndrome. Suffocation is a leading cause of death in infants, so it's crucial that you don't leave the baby unattended anywhere there is something that could suffocate them. When you place your little one on a hard surface, it will not change its form or mold to the shape of the infant's head in any way. However, if you place your baby in a prone position or they roll over to this position, soft mattresses, including those constructed from memory foam, may form a pocket-like depression at the points of impact. This depression increases the danger of your baby failing to breathe. When choosing a sleeping surface for your baby, the trick is to remember that if the mattress is too soft, there is a higher chance of suffocation.

- Always try to breastfeed the baby unless there are serious reasons not to.

From time to time, medical professionals advise that breastfeeding reduces the risk of sudden infant death syndrome occurring. The mother can either choose to only breastfeed her bundle of happiness during the first six months, or she can express milk into a bottle and bottle feed the baby instead. It is important to know that infant formula may not be the best feeding option for your baby because human milk is more beneficial and protective compared to these other supplements. You will also want to avoid other non-human milk-based supplementation at all costs because they do not have everything the baby needs.

How the Baby's Crib Should Be

As a new dad, It is important to keep soft objects such as pillows, pillow-like toys, comforters, quilts, and sheepskins away from the infant's sleeping area. This will help reduce the risk of sudden infant death syndrome (SIDS), suffocation, entrapment, and strangulation. You should also keep loose bedding, such as blankets and unfitted sheets away from your baby's sleeping area. Baby sleep gear, such as a wearable blanket, is preferable to blankets and other covers to keep your baby warm while they are sleeping. This is because when an infant wears a blanket while they are sleeping, there is no chance of the blanket entangling or covering their head while they are sleeping. Experts strongly suggest that you buy a crib, bassinet, portable crib, or play yard for your baby that satisfies the safety requirements specified by the Consumer Product

Safety Commission (CPSC). The slat spacing must be smaller than 2⅜ inches, the mattresses must be firm, and there must be no drop sides. These are some of the requirements that make up these standards. The sleeping area should be devoid of potential risks such as toys, dangling cords, electric wires, and other cushions and bedding items in order to prevent the risk of asphyxia or strangulation.

Where the Baby's Crib Should Be

It is best that babies sleep in the same room as their parents, preferably within proximity to the parents' bed, but on a different surface that is made exclusively for the little one. At the very least, you need to do this for the first six months of your baby's life, but ideally, you should do it for the entire first year. Having your little one sleep in the same room with you and your partner or each of you may reduce the baby's risk of sudden infant death syndrome. However, it is important to remember that this does not imply sleeping in the same bed as your baby because that is dangerous.

There is an increased danger of suffocation, strangling, and trapping when you let your newborn sleep in the same bed as you adults. You can reduce the risk of these dangers occurring by not sharing the same bed with your baby. It is recommended that you keep the child's bed, regardless of whether it is a stationary crib, a portable crib, a play yard, or a bassinet, in the same room as you until the little one reaches the age of one year. Even though there is no conclusive evidence to support shifting a baby into their own room before the age of one year, the first six months are very important. This is a result of the fact that the rates of SIDS and other sleep-related deaths, in particular those happening in scenarios in which individuals share a bed, are at their highest in the first six months of a baby's life. If you place the crib in such a way that it is close to the room in which you sleep, it will be much easier for the parents to feed, comfort, and otherwise keep an eye on the baby.

Chapter 8:

Advice From Father to Father

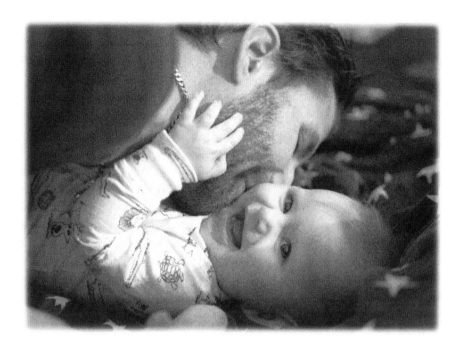

Holding the Baby Right

Your baby is here now, but do you know how to hold your newborn? This can be scary as the baby is tiny in the first few weeks. You may worry about the possibility of accidentally dropping them, twisting their body, or even breaking their fragile bones, so it is important that you learn to do it the correct way.

It's only natural for new dads to feel anxious when holding their new neonates for the first time. When holding your baby, there are a few considerations that you need to take note of. Supporting your baby's head and neck when carrying or holding him is the most crucial step. It will be your responsibility to make sure that your baby's head does not flop from side to side or snap from front to back until they are about four months old when they will begin to develop head control.

If you want to hold your baby in an upright position, you should support your baby's head and neck with one hand while holding them against your chest and shoulder. At the same time, use your other hand to support the bottom. This will ensure stability when holding your baby.

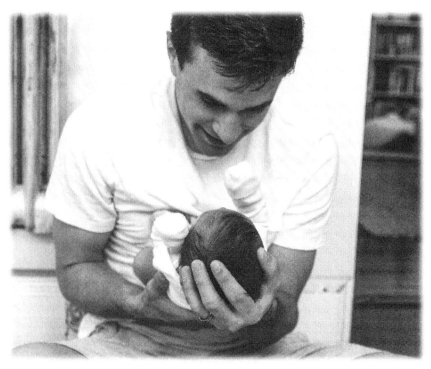

If you want to lift your baby from the crib or from a laying down position, support their head when doing so. Paying special attention to the soft depressed-like spots on the baby's skull (fontanelles). Put one hand under your baby's head and neck and the other hand under the bottoms when picking them up. To avoid arching your back, flex your knees. You should now have a firm grasp on your little one. Take the baby in your arms and bring them close to your chest as you straighten your legs.

Bathing the Baby Right

As a dad, you may want to help your partner out with bathing the baby. However, when you are scared of hurting the delicate little human by mistake, the entire idea of offering some support can give you chills. Don't be scared; let's take a quick look at how you can even become your baby's favorite person when it's time to bathe!

Pick a moment when your baby is active and awake. Ensure the room is not cold. Prepare everything in advance. You will require a dish of warm water, a towel, cotton wool, a new diaper, baby powder, lotion, and clean clothes if necessary.

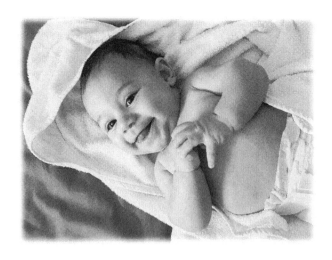

Note, you don't have to bathe your baby every day, you can bathe them 3 to 4 times per week unless when necessary. You should use warm water, not hot water. In order to prevent burning your baby, use your elbow to check the temperature of the water and thoroughly mix the water. For the first month, plain water is ideal for your baby's skin. While holding your infant on your knee, wash their face. Next, support them over the bowl or dish as you wash their hair with simple water. After gently drying their hair. With one hand supporting their head and shoulders and the other holding their upper arm, carefully lower your baby into the dish or bath. Then, without splashing, use the other hand to gently swish the water over your infant. Avoid letting your baby's head touch the water. Never, not even for a second, leave your baby unattended in the bathtub. Lift your baby out and towel them off, paying close attention to any skin folds. Your infant might benefit from a massage right now. Till your kid is at least one month old, refrain from applying any oils or lotions. Dress the baby up and make sure he keeps warm.

Determining If the Baby Feels Warm

As a new dad, you are completely new to taking care of babies and it is not in your nature yet to know if it is too hot or cold for your baby. So you probably have a lot of questions which will be covered here.

How warm does the baby's room need to be while it's cold? When summer is in full swing and it's scorching outside, how should you control your air conditioner? How can you determine whether your child is too hot or too cold?

The normal baby's temperature ranges between 98°F and 100.3°F for a normal temperature reading and 100.4°F or greater is considered a fever. The best course of action is to consult your pediatrician if your baby's temperature is elevated, especially if accompanying symptoms like a runny nose, sore throat, or cough continue.

So, without a thermometer, how would you tell if your baby is too hot or cold?

By feeling the nape of the neck to see if it is sweaty or frigid to the touch, you can determine whether your infant is too hot or too cold. If your little one feels overheated, they will sweat and their cheeks will flush. A baby that is hot might also breathe very fast. The baby may appear less active and have very chilly hands and feet If It Is too cold.

Chapter 9:

Getting Out of the House With

Your Baby

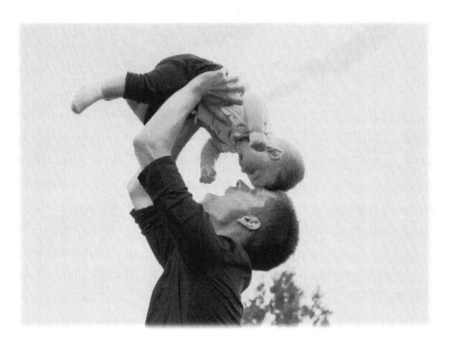

Sometimes, people think having a baby means they are stuck at home, changing diapers and trimming nails. However, the truth is you can still go out and enjoy life with your baby!

There are plenty of activities you can do outside while getting some air with your little one. Even a nature walk in the park can be a memorable way to bond with your baby and partner. Do not be afraid to explore beyond your imagination and make it more exciting.

One can safely travel without worry with an infant; however, one must take various precautions depending on the destination and the means of transportation chosen to travel.

The points listed below are some of the advice from pediatricians:

Air travel:

Healthy infants born at the right time can travel by air 48 hours after birth; however, it is preferable to wait at least one week after birth. This is because the baby is subjected to various temperature and pressure changes as well as noises and lights that can disturb its sleep.

It is advisable to stimulate feedings often as doing so reduces the possibility of the infant experiencing pain due to the change in pressure inside the plane during takeoff and landing.

In the case of premature infants and those with heart or lung disease, I strongly recommend that you seek advice from your medical professional.

Car travel:

Infants can travel by car if suitable thermal conditions can be ensured inside the passenger compartment;

however, it is preferable to wait until about a week after birth.

According to road regulations, the infant will have to travel inside the compliant "baby seat/booster seat," so if the infant is too small, it is unlikely to be placed in the correct manner.

- The car seat must mandatorily be installed in the opposite direction of travel until the infant weighs at least 9 kg. It is safer if it is installed in the rear seats; be careful not to deactivate the airbags if you install the seat in the front seat!
- The temperature inside the passenger compartment should be about 71,6 F° (22 C°).

I recommend taking a break to let the infant eat every two hours of travel.

Train travel:

Traveling by train is very comfortable since the temperature is almost always as desired, plus there is plenty of room to move around and possibly cradle your newborn, who can comfortably sit in the arms of you or your partner.

Where to go with a newborn?

It's up to you to choose the destination!

Mountain trips:

If you like the mountains, I recommend staying for medium to long periods of time because the infant's body has to get used to the atmospheric pressure of the location. Too short a stay could lead to imbalances.

Heights that exceed 6,500 ft (2,000 m) are to be avoided.

It is important to remember that infants do not have muscular or bone structures that can withstand being carried, so it is best to avoid too long walks.

Beach trips:

You must always keep in mind that the newborn baby is vulnerable to temperature changes, so I recommend going out during cooler hours and always ensuring that your baby is placed in the shade since babies' skin is not yet able to withstand direct UV rays.

Remember to breastfeed your baby often because he or she may run the risk of dehydration. You will notice this when the infant urinates very little, has dry mucous membranes, and may be irritable or extremely sleepy.

- For infants less than six months old: they should definitely wear clothes that cover most of their skin, have suitable sunscreen applied to their delicate skin often, and absolutely stay in the shade.
- For infants over six months old: apply sunscreen that protects against UVA and UVB rays and is suitable for their delicate skin; they can wear various swimsuits.

They must wear certified caps and sunglasses.

I recommend that you choose beaches or establishments that are well-equipped for children (this is a feature you will find pointed out when booking).

Trips to the countryside:

This is ideal for babies. The countryside is notoriously calm and quiet, and there is a nice, temperate climate, so it is neither too hot nor too cold. The infant will be able to have sleeping and waking rhythms, and the tranquil countryside facilitates these rhythms.

I only recommend avoiding places near stables and ponds since there are many "hematophagous" insects, i.e., insects that feed on blood and can cause diseases, even serious ones, to develop. Babies' skin will not tolerate anti-insect products.

What to pack:

Stock up on:

- wet wipes suitable for baby's delicate skin;
- plenty of diapers;
- covers to protect baby from possible air conditioning;
- bibs;
- hygiene products;
- saline solution for nasal washes;
- ointments that combat skin redness;
- sunscreens; I recommend those containing minerals such as zinc oxide or titanium that have the power to prevent the sun's rays from penetrating the skin. I also recommend that you apply sunscreen everywhere (remember that UVA and UVB rays are anywhere you are exposed to direct sunlight);
- medical kit; under the advice and prescription of your medical professional, bring a small kit of medications that can prepare you for every eventuality—from unexpected fever to diarrheal discharges.

As for the little one's clothes, they obviously depend on the destination you choose.

For the seaside or warm climates, I recommend clothing made of natural fibers to let the baby's skin breathe, light colors (to repel the sun's rays), and hats with wide brims to protect from the sun and possible conjunctivitis.

For the mountains or cold climates, of course, I recommend technical or otherwise suitable clothing so that the infant's body temperature does not drop too low.

In locations with lots of insects, be prepared! At the market, find a wide variety of mosquito nets appropriate for strollers, cribs, and beach laptops.

Conclusion

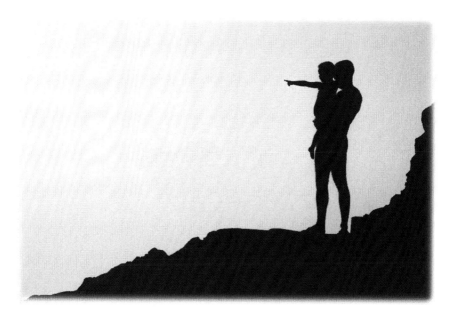

You are on the right path, dear dad-to-be. You can do this!

If you found helpful information in this book and enjoyed the read, you can help other dads learn something by sharing or recommending it to your friends.

Printed in Great Britain
by Amazon

14192644R00056